pregnancy notes

Due date . . . .

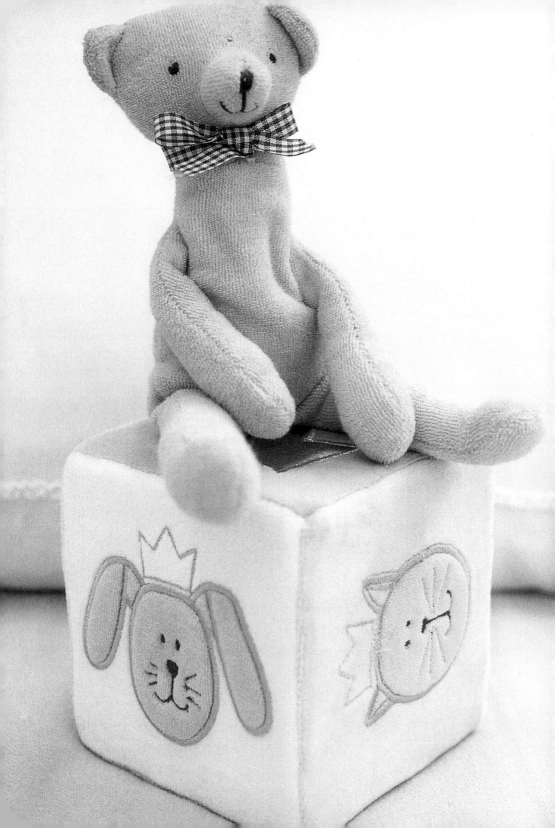

pregnancy
notes

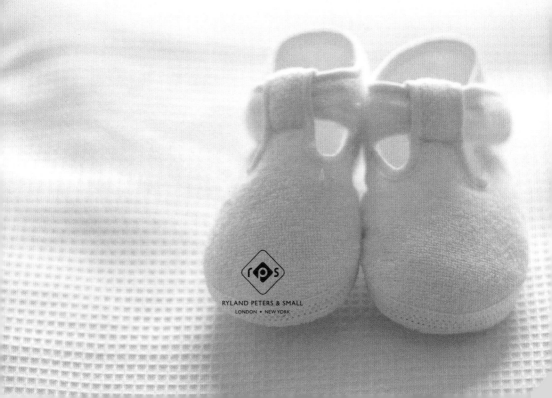

RYLAND PETERS & SMALL
LONDON • NEW YORK

Text Dawn Bates

Senior designer Julie Bennett
Commissioning editor Nathan Joyce

Head of production Patricia Harrington
Production Silvia La Greca
Art director Leslie Harrington
Editorial director Julia Charles

First published in 2014 by
Ryland Peters and Small
20–21 Jockey's Fields
London WC1R 4BW
and
519 Broadway, 5th Floor
New York, NY 10012

www.rylandpeters.com

10 9 8 7 6 5 4 3 2 1

Text, design and photographs
© Ryland Peters & Small 2014

ISBN: 978-1-84975-514-6

Printed and bound in China

While the advice and information are
believed to be true at the time of going
to press, the publisher cannot accept any
legal responsibility or liability for any
errors or omissions that may be made.
This journal is not designed to be a
comprehensive reference book on
pregnancy and the reader should always
consult a physician in all matters
relating to health and particularly in
respect of any symptoms that may
require diagnosis or medical attention.

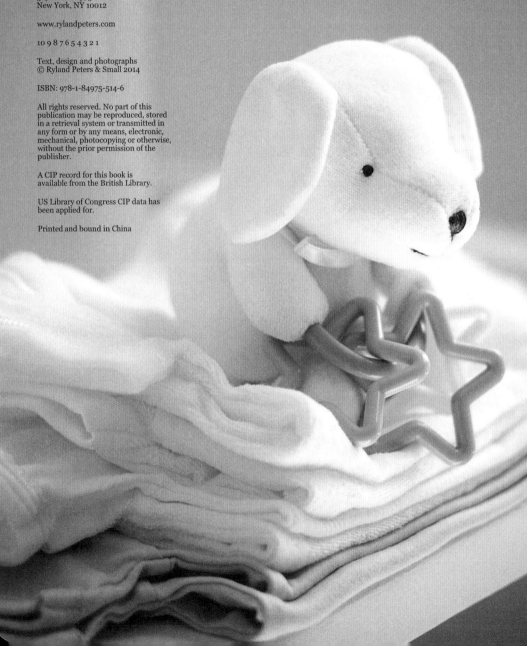

contents

Introduction	6
My Pregnancy	7
Useful Contacts	8
PREGNANCY HEALTH	**10**
My Medical History	12
Healthy Eating	14
Keeping Fit	16
Weight Monitoring	20
Antenatal Care	22
Antenatal Classes	26
PREPARING FOR YOUR BABY	**30**
Budgeting	32
Buying Equipment	34
Baby Essentials	36
Borrow and Return	38
Decorating the Nursery	40
Favourite Boys' Names	44
Favourite Girls' Names	46
Baby Shower	48
Childcare Options	52
DIARY & DATES	**54**
Year-to-view Planner	56
First Trimester	60
Second Trimester	90
Third Trimester	124

LABOUR & BIRTH	**158**
Countdown to D-Day	160
Birth Plan	162
Packing Your Hospital Bag	166
Announcing the Birth	168
Record of Your Labour	170
THE EARLY WEEKS	**174**
About My Baby	176
Gifts Received	178
Feeding Log	180
Postnatal Appointments	184
To-do List	**186**
Additional Notes	**188**
Useful Organizations	**190**
Credits	192

introduction

Congratulations, you're pregnant! This invaluable journal is designed to become your essential companion in the coming months. To ensure you and your baby stay in good health, there are sections for antenatal appointments and medical notes as well as guidance on healthy eating and keeping fit.

The wonderful week-by-week section enables you to follow your unborn baby's progress and keep a detailed record of your pregnancy. Stay organized and in control with equipment and baby essentials checklists, baby names shortlists, birth plan notes and much more. Before you know it you'll be filling in that new baby section and enjoying looking back at this incredible record of one of the most exciting times of your life.

my pregnancy

Record the details of medical personnel here and any contact details that may be needed in an emergency.

Name:

Date of birth:

Due date:

Emergency contact 1:

Telephone Number:

Emergency contact 2:

Telephone Number:

Hospital :

Labour ward telephone number:

Name of midwife:

Midwife's telephone number:

Local taxi telephone number:

useful contacts

Note down contact details and opening times here.

Doctor's surgery

Name(s):

Tel no: Email:

Address:

Opening times/availability:

Health clinic

Name(s):

Tel no: Email:

Address:

Opening times/availability:

Hospital

Name(s):

Tel no: Email:

Address:

Opening times/availability:

useful contacts

Pharmacist

Name(s):

Tel no: Email:

Address:

Opening times/availability:

Antenatal classes

Name(s):

Tel no: Email:

Address:

Opening times/availability:

Health visitor

Name(s):

Tel no:

Email:

Address:

Opening times/availability:

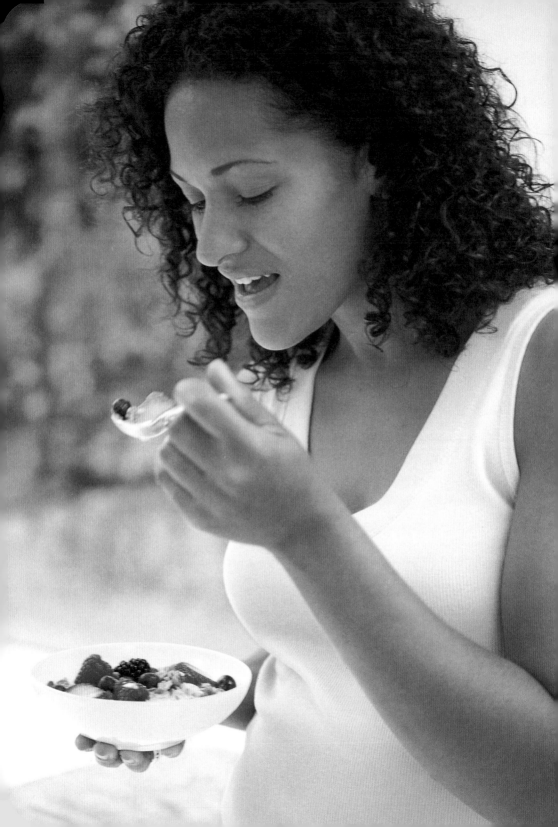

pregnancy health

Like most women, you are likely to become particularly health-conscious during pregnancy. In the following pages you can keep track of your antenatal appointments and medical care, and use the healthy eating and fitness sections to maximize your health and well-being.

my medical history

Write down important medical information here and note down any symptoms or complications of pregnancy you have experienced.

Blood group:

Immunizations:

Allergies:

Hereditary illnesses:

my medical history

Pregnancy conditions

Date	Symptoms
Doctor	Diagnosis

Treatment

Date	Symptoms
Doctor	Diagnosis

Treatment

Date	Symptoms
Doctor	Diagnosis

Treatment

Date	Symptoms
Doctor	Diagnosis

Treatment

Notes:

healthy eating

It's never been more important for you to keep track of what you're eating. Note down some healthy meal ideas here to ensure you have a balanced diet that provides all the essential nutrients for you and your growing baby.

Breakfast:

_____

_____

_____

_____

_____

_____

_____

_____

Foods to AVOID during pregnancy:
- Unpasteurized milk
- Raw or undercooked eggs
- Mould-ripened soft cheeses
- Soft blue-veined cheeses
- Pâté
- Raw or undercooked meat
- Liver or liver products
- Raw shellfish, shark, swordfish and marlin
(eat only a limited amount of other fish)

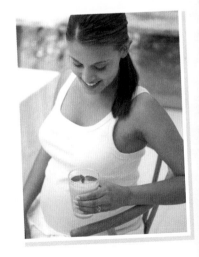

healthy eating

Lunch:

_____

_____

_____

_____

_____

Dinner:

_____

_____

_____

_____

_____

Snacks:

_____

_____

_____

_____

keeping fit

Gentle, moderate exercise is good for you and your baby. By writing down some exercise goals you're more likely to achieve them. Pelvic floor exercises are really useful during pregnancy to strengthen the muscles between your legs that support your bladder. To exercise them, sit in a comfortable position and squeeze the muscles 10–15 times. Don't hold your breath or tighten your stomach, buttock, or thigh muscles at the same time.

Week beginning

Exercise goals

Goals achieved?

Week beginning

Exercise goals

Goals achieved?

Week beginning

Exercise goals

Goals achieved?

Notes:

keeping fit

Week beginning	
Exercise goals	
Goals achieved?	

Week beginning	
Exercise goals	
Goals achieved?	

Notes:

Exercise to AVOID during your pregnancy

- Any exercise that requires you to lie flat on your back
- Contact sports
- Sports where there is a risk of falling
- Scuba-diving
- Exercise at high altitudes

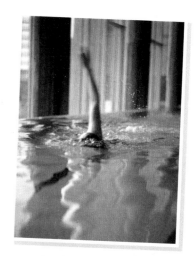

keeping fit

Week beginning	
Exercise goals	
Goals achieved?	

Week beginning	
Exercise goals	
Goals achieved?	

Week beginning	
Exercise goals	
Goals achieved?	

Notes:

keeping fit

Week beginning	
Exercise goals	
Goals achieved?	

Week beginning	
Exercise goals	
Goals achieved?	

Week beginning	
Exercise goals	
Goals achieved?	

Notes:

weight monitoring

It is both natural and healthy to gain weight during pregnancy, as your bodily systems undergo many changes to accommodate and nurture your growing baby. This is likely to be around 12.5 kg/2 stone more by the end of your pregnancy, with your baby accounting for one third of that. Keep a track of your weight gain here.

	Weight	Weight Gain		Weight	Weight Gain
Week 1			Week 17		
Week 2			Week 18		
Week 3			Week 19		
Week 4			Week 20		
Week 5			Week 21		
Week 6			Week 22		
Week 7			Week 23		
Week 8			Week 24		
Week 9			Week 25		
Week 10			Week 26		
Week 11			Week 27		
Week 12			Week 28		
Week 13			Week 29		
Week 14			Week 30		
Week 15			Week 31		
Week 16			Week 32		

weight monitoring

	Weight	Weight Gain		Weight	Weight Gain
Week 33			Week 38		
Week 34			Week 39		
Week 35			Week 40		
Week 36			Week 41		
Week 37			Week 42		

Feelings:

antenatal care

You will see the midwife by the time you are 10 weeks pregnant and then have approximately eight more appointments from week 16 onwards. Keep a note of your appointment times and write down any questions to ask.

Midwife's name:

Clinic/hospital contact details:

Week of pregnancy: Appointment date and time:

Questions to ask:

Notes:

Week of pregnancy: Appointment date and time:

Questions to ask:

Notes:

Week of pregnancy: Appointment date and time:

Questions to ask:

Notes:

antenatal care

Week of pregnancy: Appointment date and time:

Questions to ask:

Notes:

Week of pregnancy: Appointment date and time:

Questions to ask:

Notes:

Week of pregnancy: Appointment date and time:

Questions to ask:

Notes:

antenatal care

Week of pregnancy: Appointment date and time:

Questions to ask:

Notes:

Week of pregnancy: Appointment date and time:

Questions to ask:

Notes:

Week of pregnancy: Appointment date and time:

Questions to ask:

Notes:

antenatal care

Week of pregnancy: Appointment date and time:

Questions to ask:

Notes:

Week of pregnancy: Appointment date and time:

Questions to ask:

Notes:

Week of pregnancy: Appointment date and time:

Questions to ask:

Notes:

antenatal classes

Most couples attend antenatal classes in the third trimester to prepare for the birth and learn some practical parenting skills.

Location:

Antenatal teacher:

Other attendees:

Name(s)	Contact details

Date and Time of class:

Subjects covered:

Notes:

Date and Time of class:

Subjects covered:

Notes:

antenatal classes

Date and Time of class:

Subjects covered:

Notes:

Date and Time of class:

Subjects covered:

Notes:

Date and Time of class:

Subjects covered:

Notes:

Date and Time of class:

Subjects covered:

Notes:

antenatal classes

Date and Time of class:

Subjects covered:

Notes:

Date and Time of class:

Subjects covered:

Notes:

Date and Time of class:

Subjects covered:

Notes:

Date and Time of class:

Subjects covered:

Notes:

antenatal classes

Date and Time of class:

Subjects covered:

Notes:

Date and Time of class:

Subjects covered:

Notes:

Date and Time of class:

Subjects covered:

Notes:

Date and Time of class:

Subjects covered:

Notes:

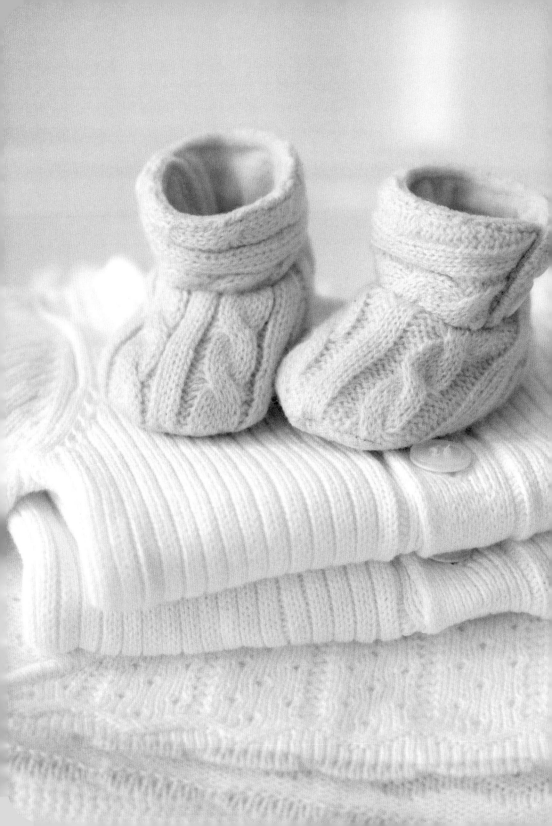

preparing for your baby

Once the initial excitement of the pregnancy test result has passed,

you will begin to turn your mind to more practical matters.

Use the pages to plan what you need to buy, note down your

favourite baby names and work out how you'll decorate the nursery.

Let someone else organize your baby shower!

budgeting

Monthly expenditure

Income after tax	
Outgoings	
Mortgage/Rent	
Utility bills	
Food	
Toiletries	
Clothing	
Travel	
Insurance	
Savings/investments	
Social life	
Debts	
Additional costs	
Total outgoings	

budgeting

Planning for baby's arrival

One-off costs	
Monthly costs	
Total costs	

Notes:

buying equipment

Your biggest expense will most likely be the equipment you'll need for your baby. Remember that you don't need everything in time for the birth so it's a good idea to stagger the cost.

	Price comparison 1	Price comparison 2	Price comparison 3
Car seat			
Moses basket			
Cot and mattress			
Pram/stroller			
Changing mat			
Changing table			
Sterilizer			
Feeding equipment			

buying equipment

	Price comparison 1	Price comparison 2	Price comparison 3
Breast pump			
Baby monitor			
Baby bath			
Baby carrier			
Bouncy chair			
Highchair			

Notes:

baby essentials

There are a few essential items your baby will need in the early weeks so buy them before your due date. Don't forget that you'll probably be given many outfits as gifts.

	Colour/style	Number purchased	Number given
Nappies/diapers			
Muslins/reusable cloths			
Sheets and bedding			
Sleeping bag			
Towels			
Long-sleeved sleepsuits			
Long-sleeved bodysuits			
Bibs			
Hat			

baby essentials

	Colour/style	Number purchased	Number given
Socks			
Cardigans			
Thermometer			
Lotions and wipes			

Notes:

borrow and return

Don't be afraid to borrow equipment and baby clothes from friends and family, particularly those with babies that have got older and outgrown their clothes! You can keep a note of who gave you each item here.

Item:

Borrowed from:

Date returned:

Item:

Borrowed from:

Date returned:

Item:

Borrowed from:

Date returned:

Item:

Borrowed from:

Date returned:

borrow and return

Item:

Borrowed from:

Date returned:

Item:

Borrowed from:

Date returned:

Item:

Borrowed from:

Date returned:

Item:

Borrowed from:

Date returned:

decorating the nursery

Getting your baby's room ready adds to the excitement and makes the idea of becoming parents seem all the more real!

Paint and wallpaper:

_____

_____

Blinds and curtains:

_____

_____

Fabrics:

_____

_____

Toys:

_____

_____

Furniture:

_____

_____

_____

_____

decorating the nursery

Other:
_____
_____
_____
_____
_____
_____
_____
_____
_____
_____
_____
_____
_____
_____
_____
_____

decorating the nursery

Stick your collected samples here:

decorating the nursery

favourite boys' names

Write your shortlist below:

Name	Meaning

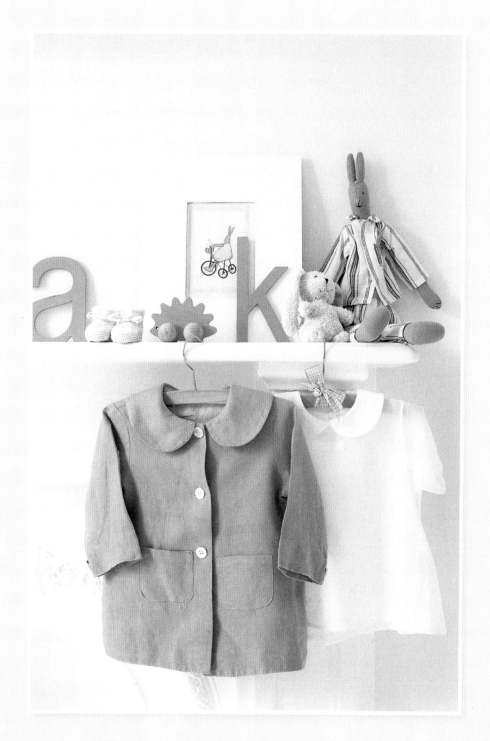

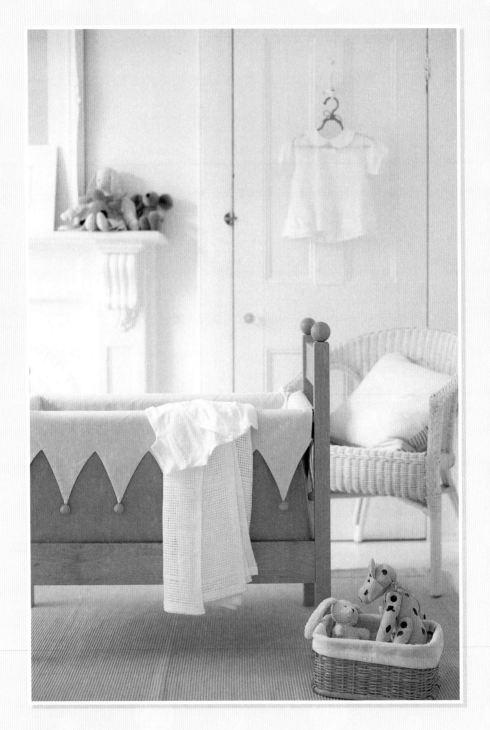

favourite girls' names

Write your shortlist below:

Name	Meaning

baby shower

Celebrate this special time with a baby shower!

Given by

Where:

When:

Guests

Name(s)	Contact details

baby shower

Gifts

From whom	Thank you card sent

Notes:

baby shower

Special messages for the baby and mum-to-be:

baby shower

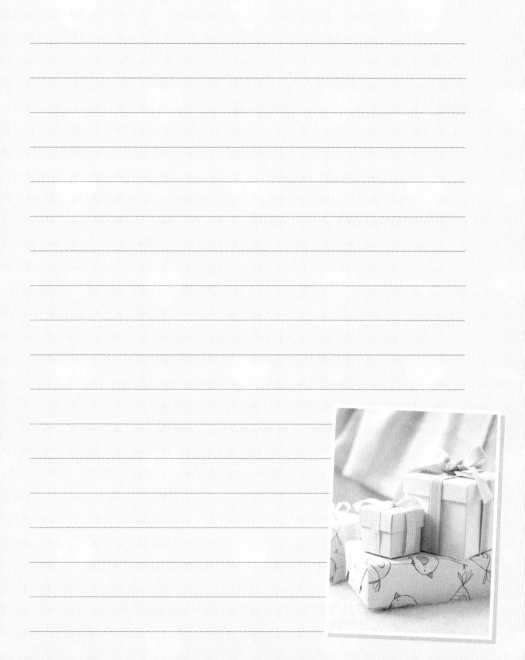

childcare options

It's worth looking into your childcare options during your pregnancy so that you have some idea of the cost involved, the availability of childminders and nannies and whether you need to go on a waiting list for a nursery.

Childminder

Name:

Contact Details:

Fees:

Availability:

Childminder

Name:

Contact Details:

Fees:

Availability:

Nursery

Name:

Contact Details:

Fees:

Availability:

childcare options

Nursery

Name:

Contact Details:

Fees:

Availability:

Nanny

Name:

Contact Details:

Fees:

Availability:

Nanny

Name:

Contact Details:

Fees:

Availability:

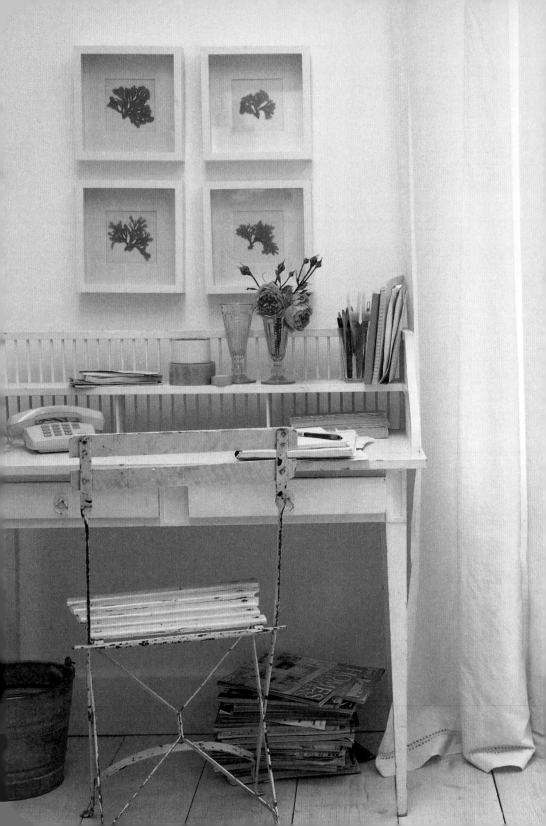

diary & dates

From now on the main focus of every week will be your pregnancy.
These pages are designed to help you follow your unborn baby's
progress and keep a record of this very special time.

year-to-view planner

	January	February	March
1			
2			
3			
4			
5			
6			
7			
8			
9			
10			
11			
12			
13			
14			
15			
16			
17			
18			
19			
20			
21			
22			
23			
24			
25			
26			
27			
28			
29			
30			
31			

year-to-view planner

	April	May	June
1			
2			
3			
4			
5			
6			
7			
8			
9			
10			
11			
12			
13			
14			
15			
16			
17			
18			
19			
20			
21			
22			
23			
24			
25			
26			
27			
28			
29			
30			
31			

year-to-view planner

	July	August	September
1			
2			
3			
4			
5			
6			
7			
8			
9			
10			
11			
12			
13			
14			
15			
16			
17			
18			
19			
20			
21			
22			
23			
24			
25			
26			
27			
28			
29			
30			
31			

year-to-view planner

	October	November	December
1			
2			
3			
4			
5			
6			
7			
8			
9			
10			
11			
12			
13			
14			
15			
16			
17			
18			
19			
20			
21			
22			
23			
24			
25			
26			
27			
28			
29			
30			
31			

1st trimester

EARLY DAYS

Although you are bound to be excited at the prospect of having a baby, the first three months are also an anxious time in any pregnancy and a time when you are probably trying to keep it a secret from most people. Your body shape shouldn't change too much over the next 14 weeks but you may be tired and nauseous. You may also be bloated and feel faint.

It's not all bad news though! Just think, this is the start of the most wonderful stage in your life so far, and your body is simply adapting to the task ahead. And in nine months' time you will have a beautiful new baby to love and cherish.

"A journey of a thousand miles must begin with a single step."

The Way of Lao Tzu, Lao Tzu (6th Century BC)

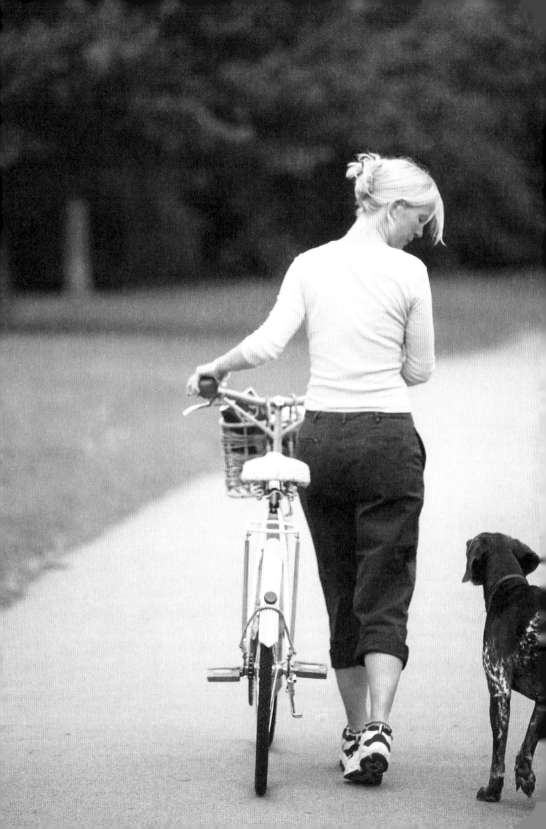

week 1

To avoid confusion over the exact day your baby is conceived, the first day of pregnancy is taken as the first day of your last period. As today is the first day of your period you won't have conceived yet, but as this is the date your pregnancy will be dated from, make a note of it here. As you are trying for a baby, you may want to buy and borrow some books on pregnancy.

Date pregnancy will be dated from:

Notes:

ADVICE when trying for a baby
- Eat a well-balanced diet.
- Take the recommended daily amount of folic acid/folate (400mcg).
- Avoid taking any drugs or medication that haven't been prescribed for you by your doctor.
- Make sure your doctor knows that there is a possibility you could be pregnant before writing a prescription.

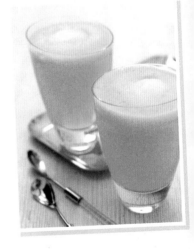

week 1

Keep a record of any pregnancy books you have borrowed:

Title:

Who borrowed from:

Title:

Who borrowed from:

Title:

Who borrowed from:

Title:

Who borrowed from:

Title:

Who borrowed from:

Title:

Who borrowed from:

week 2

As most women ovulate between 12 and 16 days before their next period, ovulation will take place towards the end of this week or the beginning of week 3.

Notes:

_____

_____

_____

_____

_____

_____

_____

_____

_____

DID YOU KNOW?

The sex of your baby is determined by your partner's sperm. However, if you do want to try for a particular sex some schools of thought recommend certain natural ways to increase your chances towards your preferred choice. According to some, it's all in your diet. The theory goes that if you want a girl you should eat starchy foods and dairy products and if it's a boy you're after you should concentrate on meat and fruit. Others say it's all in the timing – and that having sex on your ovulation day increases your chances of having a boy. There is some research that disputes this claim, but you could always buy a home ovulation kit and try it out!

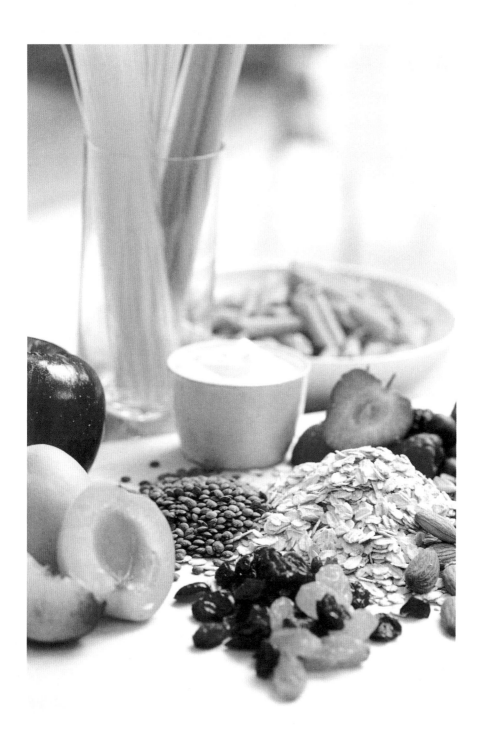

week 3

You have now conceived! Although some women say they knew they were pregnant from day one, you are unlikely to notice any hormonal changes at this early stage.

How I felt when I found out I was pregnant:

_____

_____

_____

_____

_____

_____

How my partner felt:

_____

_____

_____

_____

_____

_____

_____

_____

_____

week 3

By now you are carrying a tiny cluster of 16 cells, which are the beginnings of your baby. This new life already has a determined sex.

week 4

You may start to notice some differences at this stage in your pregnancy. Your breasts may be swollen and tender, and you may be feeling quite tired and nauseous.

How am I feeling this week?

Date:	Energy:
Mood:	Appetite:
Cravings:	Sickness:

Date:	Energy:
Mood:	Appetite:
Cravings:	Sickness:

Date:	Energy:
Mood:	Appetite:
Cravings:	Sickness:

Date:	Energy:
Mood:	Appetite:
Cravings:	Sickness:

week 4

Date:	Energy:
Mood:	Appetite:
Cravings:	Sickness:

Date:	Energy:
Mood:	Appetite:
Cravings:	Sickness:

Date:	Energy:
Mood:	Appetite:
Cravings:	Sickness:

Notes:

> *Even at this very early stage in your pregnancy your baby's major internal organs are already starting to form.*

week 5

By now you will have missed your period and will realize that you are pregnant. There are plenty of reliable home-pregnancy test kits on the market, but it's always a good idea to visit your doctor at this stage. He or she will be able to tell you the estimated due date (EDD) of your baby and talk through antenatal care and birthing options with you. You might want to start booking antenatal appointments at this point.

Antenatal appointments

Location	Date and time

week 5

You may want to start thinking about where you want to have your baby – at hospital or at home. There are a number of useful online resources and forums, like babycentre.co.uk/babycenter.com, which offer information about these choices. Make a list of the pros and cons for each below.

Hospital birth

Pros	Cons

Home birth

Pros	Cons

Your baby is already changing shape, from a hollow cluster of cells to a long narrow form.

week 6

If you decide on a hospital birth rather than a home birth, there are a few things that you'll need to think about.

CONSIDER your options
• What facilities do they have for birthing options?
• What method of antenatal care do they offer?
• How easy is it to get there from home?
• What are the routes to the hospitals like during rush hour?
• What is the parking like?

List your choice of local hospitals below and note down the pros and cons for each one

Choosing a hospital	Pros and cons

By now your growing baby will be about the size of the very end of your fingertip.

week 6

Hospital choices	Pros and cons

Notes:

week 7

By now morning sickness may be a problem. One way to try to keep this under control is to eat little and often – carry snacks like raisins and biscuits in your bag just in case you need something to eat when you are out and about.

Note here anything of interest that you read in pregnancy books and magazines:

The placenta is now starting to form and this will provide your baby with all the nutrients he needs to develop throughout the pregnancy.

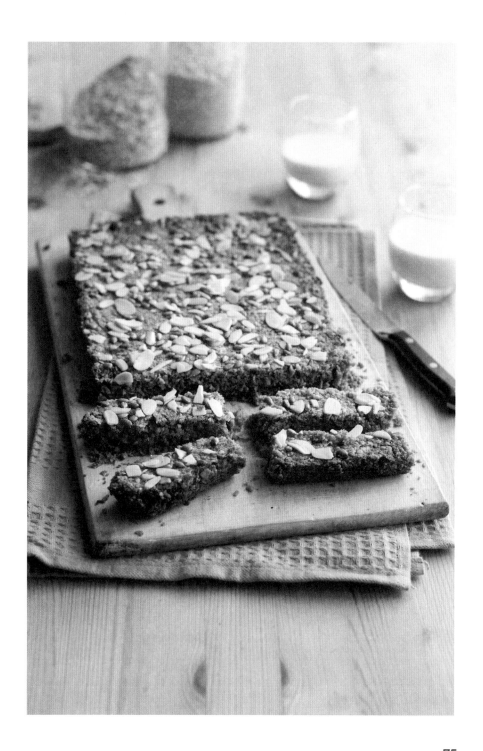

week 8

As well as feeling nauseous you may also be feeling very tired and lethargic right now. This is because your heart rate rises and your metabolic rate increases. Try to rest as much as possible, and take comfort in the fact that these feelings – both the tiredness and the nausea – should ease up in the second trimester.

How am I feeling this week?

Date:	Energy:
Mood:	Appetite:
Cravings:	Sickness:

Date:	Energy:
Mood:	Appetite:
Cravings:	Sickness:

Date:	Energy:
Mood:	Appetite:
Cravings:	Sickness:

Date:	Energy:
Mood:	Appetite:
Cravings:	Sickness:

week 8

Date:	Energy:
Mood:	Appetite:
Cravings:	Sickness:
Date:	Energy:
Mood:	Appetite:
Cravings:	Sickness:
Date:	Energy:
Mood:	Appetite:
Cravings:	Sickness:

Notes:

Your baby will now have eyes, although her eyelids will be closed over them. She will also have arms that bend at the elbows, legs that bend at the knees, and her toes will be forming.

week 9

Your skin may start to look different now. Pregnancy can cause your skin texture to change so you might need to start using different skin products, especially moisturizers.

How am I feeling this week?

Date:	Energy:
Mood:	Appetite:
Cravings:	Sickness:
Date:	Energy:
Mood:	Appetite:
Cravings:	Sickness:
Date:	Energy:
Mood:	Appetite:
Cravings:	Sickness:
Date:	Energy:
Mood:	Appetite:
Cravings:	Sickness:

week 9

Date:	Energy:
Mood:	Appetite:
Cravings:	Sickness:
Date:	Energy:
Mood:	Appetite:
Cravings:	Sickness:
Date:	Energy:
Mood:	Appetite:
Cravings:	Sickness:

Notes:

By now the placenta is fully functioning and the basic structure of all your baby's major organs is in place.

week 10

By now you may have noticed a change in your body shape – although it certainly won't be dramatic. Try to take gentle, regular exercise throughout your pregnancy.

Note down details of aquanatal classes at your local swimming pool:

Location	Time	Cost

Find out your local exercise class options and list them below:

Location	Class name	Time	Cost

Your baby's weight is now equivalent to that of a large strawberry.

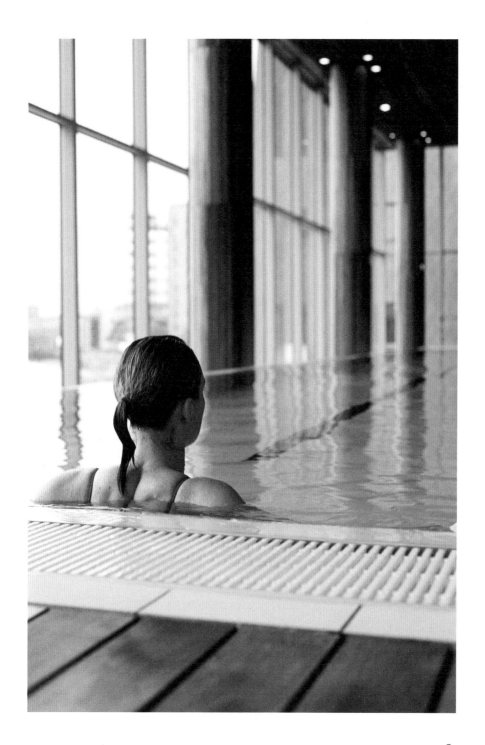

week 11

You may find that your gums are starting to bleed when you brush your teeth. It's a good idea to visit your dentist for advice on keeping your teeth healthy during your pregnancy. Make sure he knows you are expecting as some treatments, such as X-rays, are not advisable during pregnancy.

How am I feeling this week?

Date:	Energy:
Mood:	Appetite:
Cravings:	Sickness:
Date:	Energy:
Mood:	Appetite:
Cravings:	Sickness:
Date:	Energy:
Mood:	Appetite:
Cravings:	Sickness:
Date:	Energy:
Mood:	Appetite:
Cravings:	Sickness:

week 11

Date:	Energy:
Mood:	Appetite:
Cravings:	Sickness:

Date:	Energy:
Mood:	Appetite:
Cravings:	Sickness:

Date:	Energy:
Mood:	Appetite:
Cravings:	Sickness:

Notes:

Your baby is now beginning to suck, swallow and yawn.

week 12

At some point around now you may be offered a 12-week scan and your pregnancy will be dated more accurately. This will be the first time you and your partner will see your baby.

How did I feel before having the scan?

_____

_____

_____

_____

_____

_____

Stick your scan photo here

week 12

How did I feel when I saw the scan?

How did my partner feel?

At just 12 weeks all the major organs are fully formed, although your baby is still only about 6 cm (2½in) long.

first trimester round-up

Feelings:

_____

_____

_____

_____

_____

_____

_____

_____

_____

_____

_____

_____

_____

_____

_____

_____

_____

_____

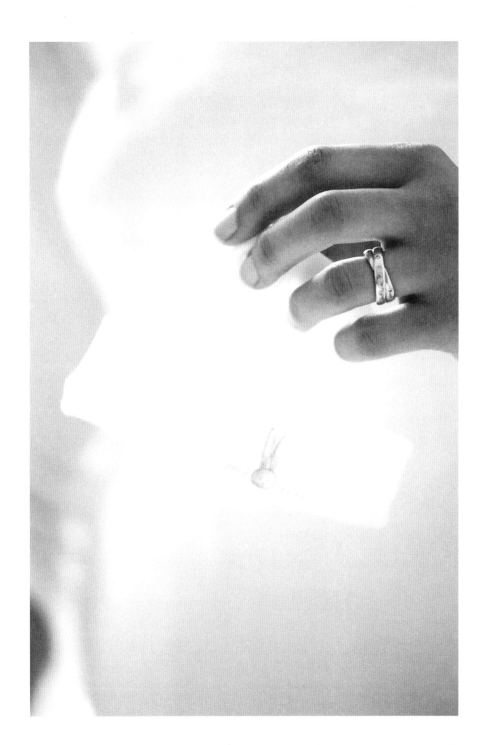

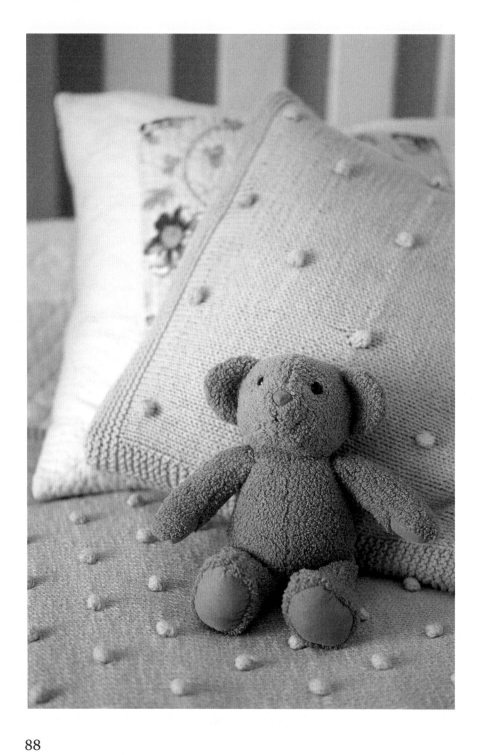

first trimester round-up

Notes:

_____

_____

_____

_____

_____

_____

_____

_____

_____

_____

_____

_____

_____

_____

2nd trimester

NEARLY HALFWAY THERE

You've reached the second trimester! This will probably be the most enjoyable part of your pregnancy. The morning sickness should ease off and your energy should return. Take advantage of this time to go out with friends, spend time with your partner and generally have some fun.

This is also an exciting time as your bump will really start to develop – and at around 18–20 weeks you will start to feel your baby moving around. Be sure to record the first time you feel him kick, not forgetting the first time you get offered a seat on public transport!

"A baby is an inestimable blessing."

Mark Twain (1835–1910)

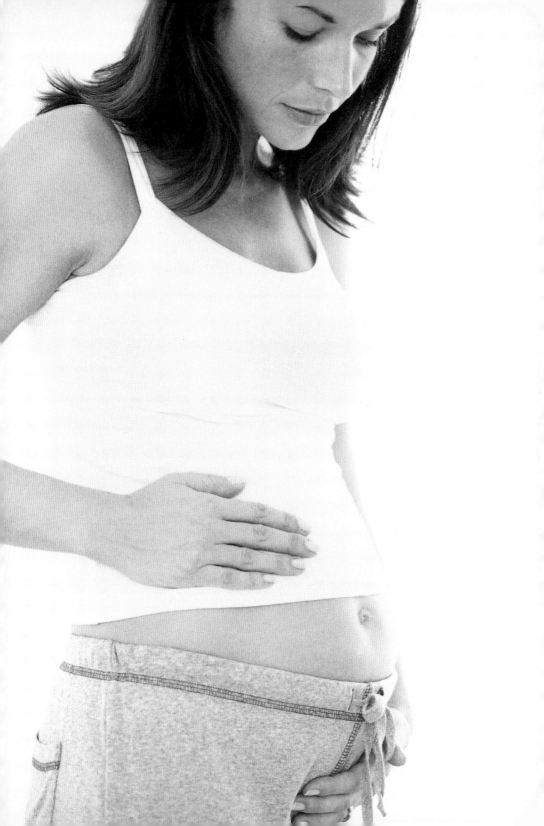

week 13

From now on your body will begin changing quite dramatically as your baby grows in size. You might want to start keeping a week-by-week photographic record of your changing body shape. The easiest way to do this is to get someone to take profile shots of you with a Polaroid or digital camera. The series of photographs will be a fascinating record that you can look back on in the years to come.

How am I feeling this week?

Date:	Energy:
Mood:	Appetite:
Cravings:	Sickness:
Date:	Energy:
Mood:	Appetite:
Cravings:	Sickness:
Date:	Energy:
Mood:	Appetite:
Cravings:	Sickness:
Date:	Energy:
Mood:	Appetite:
Cravings:	Sickness:

week 13

Date:	Energy:
Mood:	Appetite:
Cravings:	Sickness:
Date:	Energy:
Mood:	Appetite:
Cravings:	Sickness:
Date:	Energy:
Mood:	Appetite:
Cravings:	Sickness:

Notes:

Your baby now weighs about as much as a large coin. If your baby is a girl, her ovaries will now contain approximately 2 million eggs – all the eggs she'll ever have.

week 14

Once you have had your first scan and know all is well, you might want to start telling your friends and family your exciting news. Make a list below of all the people you want to tell and their respective reactions.

Name:

Reaction:

Name:

Reaction:

Name:

Reaction:

Name:

Reaction:

Name:

Reaction:

At this stage of pregancy, your baby's toenails and fingernails will start developing.

week 14

Name:

Reaction:

Name:

Reaction:

Name:

Reaction:

Name:

Reaction:

Notes:

week 15

Your sickness may have completely eased off by now, although with your expanding waistline you're probably having trouble getting into some of your clothes.

IDEAS for maternity clothing
• Choose items that are a couple of sizes larger than usual.
• Elasticated and drawstring trousers are a good option at this stage.
• Don't buy everything at once while your body shape is changing.
• See if you can borrow any maternity clothes from friends or family.

Items bought/borrowed	From where/whom

week 15

Items bought/borrowed	From where/whom

Notes:

Your baby will now fit into the palm of your hand.

week 16

If you haven't done so already, check out the situation with regards to your local antenatal or parentcraft classes. Make a list of all the ones that are available in your area and then work out which ones you would like to sign up for.

Class	Contact Details	Start Date	End Date

How am I feeling this week?

Date: Energy/Mood:

Cravings/Appetite: Health:

Notes:

By now your baby is very active and can suck her thumb and make a fist.

week 16

Date:	Energy/Mood:
Cravings/Appetite:	Health:

Date:	Energy/Mood:
Cravings/Appetite:	Health:

Date:	Energy/Mood:
Cravings/Appetite:	Health:

Date:	Energy/Mood:
Cravings/Appetite:	Health:

Date:	Energy/Mood:
Cravings/Appetite:	Health:

Date:	Energy/Mood:
Cravings/Appetite:	Health:

week 17

A dark line may appear down the centre of your abdomen at this stage in your pregnancy, called the linea nigra. It marks the division of your abdominal muscles, which separate slightly in order to make room for your expanding uterus. You might want to continue keeping a photographic record of your changing body shape.

How am I feeling this week?

Date:	Energy:
Mood:	Appetite:
Cravings:	Sickness:
Date:	Energy:
Mood:	Appetite:
Cravings:	Sickness:
Date:	Energy:
Mood:	Appetite:
Cravings:	Sickness:
Date:	Energy:
Mood:	Appetite:
Cravings:	Sickness:

week 17

Date:	Energy:
Mood:	Appetite:
Cravings:	Sickness:

Date:	Energy:
Mood:	Appetite:
Cravings:	Sickness:

Date:	Energy:
Mood:	Appetite:
Cravings:	Sickness:

Notes:

There's a small possibility you will be able to feel your baby's movements, but don't worry if you can't feel him yet — it can happen much later, especially if you're a first-time mum.

week 18

You may have started having quite vivid dreams, although this may occur later in pregnancy for some women. Try to remember them when you wake up and write them down in a dream diary or just jot them down in your journal notes – it will make for interesting reading later on.

Dream diary entry:

_____

_____

_____

Dream diary entry:

_____

_____

_____

_____

Dream diary entry:

_____

_____

_____

DID YOU KNOW?
When your baby is born he will have 300 bones in his body. However, as he grows up some of them will fuse together so by the time he reaches adulthood he will have just 206 bones.

week 18

Dream diary entry:

_____

_____

_____

Dream diary entry:

_____

_____

_____

Dream diary entry:

_____

_____

Notes:

_____

_____

_____

Your baby's eyes are now sensitive to light and his eye muscles are strong enough to move them from side to side while looking down. He will also be able to hear loud noises, although he will be unable to interpret them until the third trimester.

week 19

You may be having your fetal anomaly scan next week. This is a serious diagnostic tool that enables the radiographer to check for any development or growth problems your baby may be experiencing. The radiographer may also be able to tell you your baby's sex at this stage, should you wish to know.

Do we want to know our baby's sex?

Pros	Cons

How am I feeling this week?

Date:	Energy:
Mood:	Appetite:
Cravings:	Sickness:

Date:	Energy:
Mood:	Appetite:
Cravings:	Sickness:

Date:	Energy:
Mood:	Appetite:
Cravings:	Sickness:

week 19

Date:	Energy:
Mood:	Appetite:
Cravings:	Sickness:

Date:	Energy:
Mood:	Appetite:
Cravings:	Sickness:

Date:	Energy:
Mood:	Appetite:
Cravings:	Sickness:

Date:	Energy:
Mood:	Appetite:
Cravings:	Sickness:

Your baby's head is now about one third of the size of her body.

week 20

Before you go for the fetal anomaly scan, talk to your midwife about exactly what the scan will be checking, and the accuracy of the measurements. Make a note of any anxieties or questions you have about the results of the scan, and possible consequences for you and your baby.

Questions I would like to ask when I attend the scan:

_____

_____

_____

_____

Stick your scan photo here:

week 20

How am I feeling about the scan?

_____

_____

_____

_____

_____

_____

_____

How is my partner feeling?

_____

_____

_____

_____

_____

_____

At 20 weeks your baby's first teeth will have developed in her gums.

week 21

Your weight will have been gradually increasing throughout your pregnancy and you will have been gaining weight steadily from about week 12. Most women put on between 6–19 kg (1–3 stone) during their pregnancy. Although your appetite will also be increasing, you don't actually need to eat for two! Due to a change in your metabolism your body needs only an extra 500 calories a day to support your pregnancy. You should never diet during pregnancy, except under doctor's orders.

How am I feeling this week?

Date:	Energy:
Mood:	Appetite:
Cravings:	Health:
Date:	Energy:
Mood:	Appetite:
Cravings:	Health:
Date:	Energy:
Mood:	Appetite:
Cravings:	Health:

All of your baby's fingers are now fully formed and she has developed the ability to grasp.

week 21

Date:	Energy:
Mood:	Appetite:
Cravings:	Health:

Date:	Energy:
Mood:	Appetite:
Cravings:	Health:

Date:	Energy:
Mood:	Appetite:
Cravings:	Health:

Date:	Energy:
Mood:	Appetite:
Cravings:	Health:

Notes:

week 22

How exciting – you are now over halfway there! This is a good time to start thinking about decorating the nursery – although if there's any painting to be done get your partner to do it as the fumes might make you feel sick or give you a headache. Many people opt for a neutral colour, especially if they don't know the sex of their baby.

How am I feeling this week?

Date:	Energy:
Mood:	Appetite:
Cravings:	Health:

Date:	Energy:
Mood:	Appetite:
Cravings:	Health:

Date:	Energy:
Mood:	Appetite:
Cravings:	Health:

Date:	Energy:
Mood:	Appetite:
Cravings:	Health:

week 22

Date: | Energy:

Mood: | Appetite:

Cravings: | Health:

Date: | Energy:

Mood: | Appetite:

Cravings: | Health:

Date: | Energy:

Mood: | Appetite:

Cravings: | Health:

Notes:

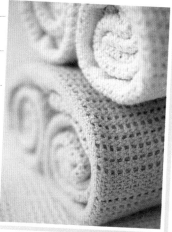

Your baby's hearing will now be acute and, although sounds will be muffled by the amniotic fluid, loud noises could make him jump.

week 23

Due to the hormonal changes you are experiencing, you may be having problems with your eyes – for example your contact lenses may be more uncomfortable than usual because your eyes are drier. These problems are only temporary, but if you do wear glasses, it's a good idea to visit your optician for a check-up.

How am I feeling this week?

Date:	Energy:
Mood:	Appetite:
Cravings:	Health:

Date:	Energy:
Mood:	Appetite:
Cravings:	Health:

Date:	Energy:
Mood:	Appetite:
Cravings:	Health:

Date:	Energy:
Mood:	Appetite:
Cravings:	Health:

week 23

Date:	Energy:
Mood:	Appetite:
Cravings:	Health:

Date:	Energy:
Mood:	Appetite:
Cravings:	Health:

Date:	Energy:
Mood:	Appetite:
Cravings:	Health:

Notes:

This week your baby's eyelids will open, but he/she won't be able to see much because your uterus is dark (although it will get lighter as your skin stretches). Her visual range will be limited until a few weeks after birth.

week 24

Your energy levels should have risen considerably so it would be a good time to do some shopping in preparation for your new arrival or to catch up with friends. By now, your baby's nervous system and muscles will have developed enough to enable her to move around inside you. The first time you feel her making small movements will be an exhilarating experience. Make a note below of how it feels.

What does the sensation feel like?

Does the baby stop kicking when your partner touches your tummy?

How am I feeling this week?

Date:	Energy:
Mood:	Appetite:
Cravings:	Health:
Date:	Energy:
Mood:	Appetite:
Cravings:	Health:
Date:	Energy:
Mood:	Appetite:
Cravings:	Health:

week 24

Date:	Energy:
Mood:	Appetite:
Cravings:	Health:

Date:	Energy:
Mood:	Appetite:
Cravings:	Health:

Date:	Energy:
Mood:	Appetite:
Cravings:	Health:

Date:	Energy:
Mood:	Appetite:
Cravings:	Health:

With the exception of the lungs, all your baby's major organs are now functioning. All the facial features are formed too.

week 25

If you fancy one last trip abroad before you've got your hands full, now's the time to do it. You have higher energy levels than you've had in a while, you won't be too large and cumbersome yet, and most importantly the airlines are still willing to let you on board! If you want to fly after 28 weeks, it's best to check with the airline.

FLYING when pregnant
• After 28 weeks, airlines will require a doctor's certificate, and some may refuse to take you.
• Most airlines will not let you on board after 34 weeks.
• Check that you're covered by your travel insurance for flying when you're in the latter stages of pregnancy.

How am I feeling this week?

Date:	Energy:
Mood:	Appetite:
Cravings:	Health:

Date:	Energy:
Mood:	Appetite:
Cravings:	Health:

Date:	Energy:
Mood:	Appetite:
Cravings:	Health:

week 25

Date:	Energy:
Mood:	Appetite:
Cravings:	Health:

Date:	Energy:
Mood:	Appetite:
Cravings:	Health:

Date:	Energy:
Mood:	Appetite:
Cravings:	Health:

Date:	Energy:
Mood:	Appetite:
Cravings:	Health:

By now, the cells in your baby's brain responsible for promoting conscious thought are developing.

week 26

Increased movements from your baby may be stopping you from sleeping properly at night-time, especially as in many cases a baby is much more active at night time. Make sure you grab some sleep whenever you can, as you should try to get plenty of rest.

ADVICE for your well-being
• Make sure you do your pelvic floor exercises regularly to prevent stress incontinence.

How am I feeling this week?

Date:	Energy:
Mood:	Appetite:
Cravings:	Health:
Date:	Energy:
Mood:	Appetite:
Cravings:	Health:
Date:	Energy:
Mood:	Appetite:
Cravings:	Health:

Your baby's nostrils have started to open and he will make breathing movements in preparation for his first intake of air.

week 26

Date:	Energy:
Mood:	Appetite:
Cravings:	Health:

Date:	Energy:
Mood:	Appetite:
Cravings:	Health:

Date:	Energy:
Mood:	Appetite:
Cravings:	Health:

Date:	Energy:
Mood:	Appetite:
Cravings:	Health:

Notes:

second trimester round-up

Feelings:

_____

_____

_____

_____

_____

_____

_____

_____

_____

_____

_____

_____

_____

_____

_____

_____

_____

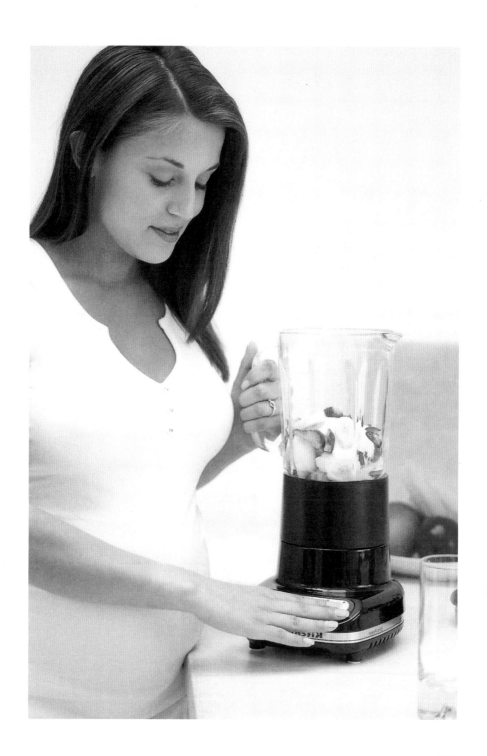

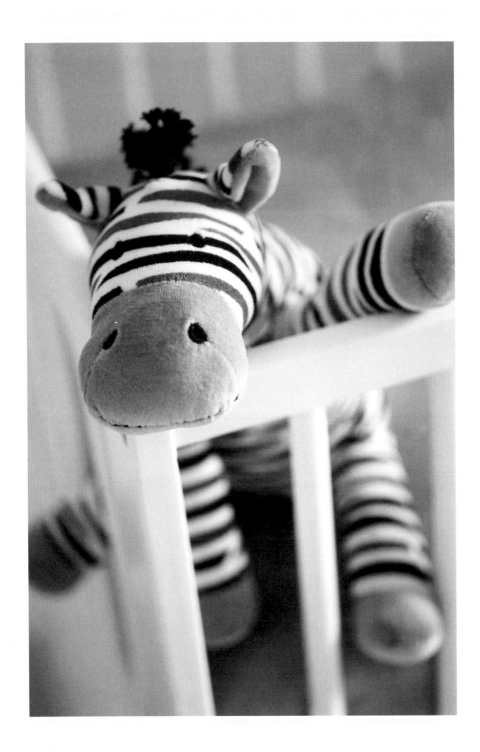

second trimester round-up

Notes:

3rd trimester

THE HOME STRETCH

You're into the third trimester and well over halfway through your pregnancy. You may start feeling like you've been pregnant forever – indeed you probably can't remember life before pregnancy! The sheer size of your bump will make it hard for you to do things towards the end of this trimester – making you short of breath, tired and preventing you from getting a good night's sleep. Grab naps where and when you can.

It's time to make sure you, your partner and your home are ready for the new arrival. Preparing for your baby as much as possible now will stop you worrying about not being ready for him when when he is finally born. Spend time going to baby shops with your partner and choose a special toy to welcome your baby into the world.

"The most effective kind of education is that a child should play amongst lovely things."

Plato (c. 429–347 BC)

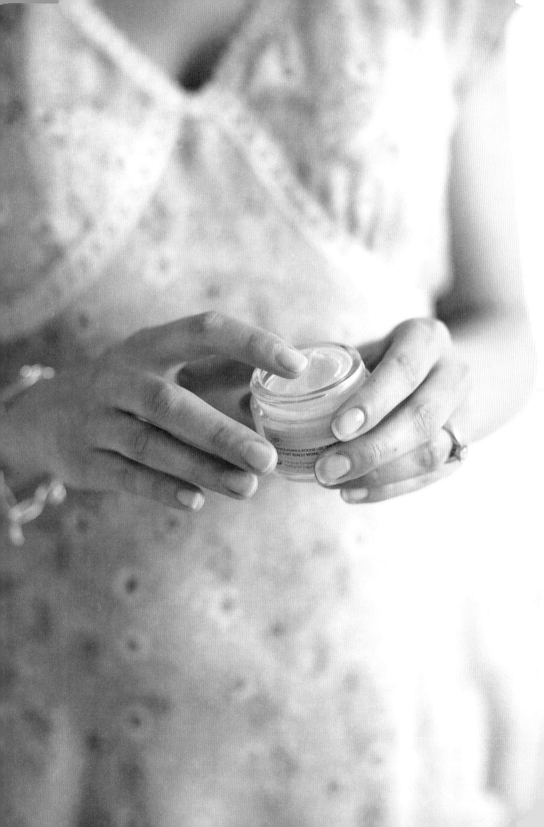

week 27

As your bump becomes more pronounced you may get increasingly bad backache. There are several things you can try to reduce its severity.

ADVICE for your backache

• Keep an eye on your posture. Don't be tempted to arch your back and don't slouch – this will only make it worse.
• Get your partner to give you a massage using a few drops of essential oil mixed with a carrier oil. Roman Camomile, Citrus, Geranium and Lavender are recommended for use in pregnancy. If you are not sure whether an oil is safe for you to use, check first with a qualified aromatherapist.
• Avoiding lifting any heavy weights if you can. If you do need to lift something, bend your knees keeping your back as straight as you can. Lift the object by straightening your legs so that your muscles do the work, not your back.

How am I feeling this week?

Date:	Energy:
Mood:	Appetite:
Date:	Energy:
Mood:	Appetite:
Date:	Energy:
Mood:	Appetite:

week 27

Date:	Energy:
Mood:	Appetite:

Date:	Energy:
Mood:	Appetite:

Date:	Energy:
Mood:	Appetite:

Date:	Energy:
Mood:	Appetite:

Notes:

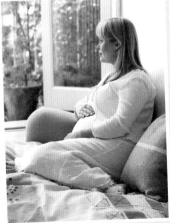

Although she is growing rapidly, your baby still only weighs 1 kg (2.2 lb) or under — just as much as a small bag of sugar.

week 28

You are now on the home straight – the third trimester – and you should be feeling fantastic, but take care not to overdo it. Spend some of each day relaxing with your feet up. This will help to relieve stress and make you less likely to suffer from swollen feet and ankles – a common complaint during pregnancy. Your hair should look and feel thicker and healthier, so it's a good time to go to the hairdressers and get an easy-to-manage hairstyle.

How am I feeling this week?

Date:	Energy:
Mood:	Appetite:
Cravings:	Health:

Date:	Energy:
Mood:	Appetite:
Cravings:	Health:

Date:	Energy:
Mood:	Appetite:
Cravings:	Health:

Date:	Energy:
Mood:	Appetite:
Cravings:	Health:

week 28

Date:	Energy:
Mood:	Appetite:
Cravings:	Health:

Date:	Energy:
Mood:	Appetite:
Cravings:	Health:

Date:	Energy:
Mood:	Appetite:
Cravings:	Health:

Notes:

Your baby is now aware of some external light.

week 29

As you start winding down at work, make sure you have your maternity benefits sorted out. Even if you are working until close to your due date, it's important to have applied for all your benefits as early as possible as it's the last thing you need to worry about once you go on maternity leave.

How am I feeling this week?

Date:	Energy:
Mood:	Appetite:
Cravings:	Health:

Date:	Energy:
Mood:	Appetite:
Cravings:	Health:

Date:	Energy:
Mood:	Appetite:
Cravings:	Health:

Date:	Energy:
Mood:	Appetite:
Cravings:	Health:

week 29

Date:	Energy:
Mood:	Appetite:
Cravings:	Health:

Date:	Energy:
Mood:	Appetite:
Cravings:	Health:

Date:	Energy:
Mood:	Appetite:
Cravings:	Health:

Notes:

Your baby now has eyelashes on her eyelids.

week 30

By this stage you probably have the impression you've been pregnant forever and may be feeling a bit fed up. Make sure you talk to your partner about how you're feeling so you don't end up arguing over petty things.

MAKING PLANS for the birth
• Start thinking about what you want to include in your birth plan.
• Discuss your options with your friends who have already had children.

How am I feeling this week?

Date:	Energy:
Mood:	Appetite:
Cravings:	Health:
Date:	Energy:
Mood:	Appetite:
Cravings:	Health:
Date:	Energy:
Mood:	Appetite:
Cravings:	Health:

Notes:

week 30

Date:	Energy:
Mood:	Appetite:
Cravings:	Health:

Date:	Energy:
Mood:	Appetite:
Cravings:	Health:

Date:	Energy:
Mood:	Appetite:
Cravings:	Health:

Date:	Energy:
Mood:	Appetite:
Cravings:	Health:

Your baby is weeing around a pint of urine a day, which your kidneys are recycling!

week 31

You may be suffering from cramps in your calf – especially during the night. There are a number of ways you can try to prevent this from happening, but if symptoms continue consult your midwife or doctor.

COPING with cramp
• Avoid wearing heels if you can: wearing flat shoes will stop your calf muscles getting bunched up.
• Relieve cramp by gently massaging the affected area.
• Stretch the muscle by flexing your foot and pushing into your heel.
• Cramp can be caused by mineral imbalances. Check with your doctor before you start taking supplements.

How am I feeling this week?

Date:	Energy:
Mood:	Appetite:
Cravings:	Health:
Date:	Energy:
Mood:	Appetite:
Cravings:	Health:
Date:	Energy:
Mood:	Appetite:
Cravings:	Health:

week 31

Date:	Energy:
Mood:	Appetite:
Cravings:	Health:

Date:	Energy:
Mood:	Appetite:
Cravings:	Health:

Date:	Energy:
Mood:	Appetite:
Cravings:	Health:

Date:	Energy:
Mood:	Appetite:
Cravings:	Health:

Your baby's growth will start to slow down between now and his birth but he will continue gaining weight.

week 32

You may be feeling practice contractions – called Braxton Hicks contractions. Most women experience these during the last few months of pregnancy. You will feel your bump tighten for about 30 seconds and this can happen a few times a day. These contractions mean your uterus is practising for the strong contractions needed in labour, but don't worry, they don't mean you are about to go into real labour.

THINGS to do
• Start thinking about ordering some of the items you will need as soon as your baby arrives.
• Bear in mind that some larger products may take up to six weeks to be delivered.

How am I feeling this week?

Date:	Energy:
Mood:	Appetite:
Cravings:	Health:

Date:	Energy:
Mood:	Appetite:
Cravings:	Health:

Date:	Energy:
Mood:	Appetite:
Cravings:	Health:

week 32

Date:	Energy:
Mood:	Appetite:
Cravings:	Health:

Date:	Energy:
Mood:	Appetite:
Cravings:	Health:

Date:	Energy:
Mood:	Appetite:
Cravings:	Health:

Date:	Energy:
Mood:	Appetite:
Cravings:	Health:

By now your baby's lungs will have developed most of their airways and air sacs ready to use after birth.

week 33

As your baby moves you will sometimes be able to see the outline of a little fist or foot in your abdomen. Share such experiences with your partner so he feels as involved in your baby's development as you are.

THINGS to do
• This is a good time to pack your hospital bag.
• If you have opted for a home birth, you'll need to prepare everything you'll need for when you go into labour.

How am I feeling this week?

Date:	Energy:
Mood:	Appetite:
Cravings:	Health:

Date:	Energy:
Mood:	Appetite:
Cravings:	
Health:	

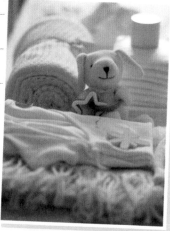

Your baby's chest movements may cause her to hiccup occasionally. You will feel these as regular little jumps.

week 33

Date:	Energy:
Mood:	Appetite:
Cravings:	Health:
Date:	Energy:
Mood:	Appetite:
Cravings:	Health:
Date:	Energy:
Mood:	Appetite:
Cravings:	Health:
Date:	Energy/Mood:
Cravings/Appetite:	Health:
Date:	Energy/Mood:
Cravings/Appetite:	Health:

week 34

For a few women, morning sickness may return at this late stage in pregnancy. If you are still at work but need to take time off as a result of pregnancy-related illness, your employer can insist that you start your maternity leave straight away. If there has been any concern about the position or size of your baby, you may have a further scan this week to check that all is well.

How am I feeling this week?

Date:	Energy:
Mood:	Appetite:
Cravings:	Health:
Date:	Energy:
Mood:	Appetite:
Cravings:	Health:
Date:	Energy:
Mood:	Appetite:
Cravings:	Health:
Date:	Energy:
Mood:	Appetite:
Cravings:	Health:

week 34

Date:	Energy:
Mood:	Appetite:
Cravings:	Health:
Date:	Energy:
Mood:	Appetite:
Cravings:	Health:
Date:	Energy:
Mood:	Appetite:
Cravings:	Health:

Notes:

By this time your baby may well be positioned with his head down so he's in the right position ready for birth.

week 35

Your size, discomfort and overall pregnant feeling may be making you feel less than attractive. Make sure you take the time to let your partner know how you're feeling so he can reassure you.

THINGS to do
• Make a list of all the people you will want to inform once your new arrival is finally here.
• Write out or use a computer to print off some name and address labels in preparation for the announcements.

How am I feeling this week?

Date:	Energy:
Mood:	Appetite:
Cravings:	Health:

Date:	Energy:
Mood:	Appetite:
Cravings:	Health:

Date:	Energy:
Mood:	Appetite:
Cravings:	Health:

week 35

Date:	Energy:
Mood:	Appetite:
Cravings:	Health:

Date:	Energy:
Mood:	Appetite:
Cravings:	Health:

Date:	Energy/Mood:
Cravings/Appetite:	Health:

Date:	Energy/Mood:
Cravings/Appetite:	Health:

With the weight your baby has gained, she is starting to run out of room in your uterus. If her squirming is bothering you, try having a long bath to make yourself more comfortable.

week 36

You may have stopped working by now and be relaxing at home. Spend lots of time pampering yourself, so you are as relaxed as possible when D-day arrives. This is also a good time to buy any last-minute items you think you might need for the birth or the nursery.

THINGS to do
• Consider hiring a TENS (Transcutaneous Electrical Nerve Stimulation) machine for pain-relief during labour. Large pharmacies hire them out. Book and collect the machine in advance to give you time to familiarize yourself with how it works.

How am I feeling this week?

Date:	Energy:
Mood:	Appetite:
Cravings:	Health:

Date:	Energy:
Mood:	Appetite:
Cravings:	Health:

Date:	Energy:
Mood:	Appetite:
Cravings:	Health:

week 36

Date:	Energy:
Mood:	Appetite:
Cravings:	Health:

Date:	Energy:
Mood:	Appetite:
Cravings:	Health:

Date:	Energy:
Mood:	Appetite:
Cravings:	Health:

Date:	Energy:
Mood:	Appetite:
Cravings:	Health:

At this point your baby's fingernails and toenails are fully grown.

week 37

You are nearly there! However, 95 per cent of healthy babies are born on days other than their due date – generally within a fortnight of the estimated date – so get ready, your baby could be coming any time now.

THINGS to do
• Make sure you have a fully stocked freezer and kitchen cupboards.
• Make some meals in advance, if possible, and freeze them.

Make a list of all the essentials food items below:

_____

_____

_____

_____

How am I feeling this week?

Date:	Energy/Mood:
Cravings/Appetite:	Health:
Date:	Energy/Mood:
Cravings/Appetite:	Health:
Date:	Energy/Mood:
Cravings/Appetite:	Health:

week 37

Date:	Energy/Mood:
Cravings/Appetite:	Health:

Date:	Energy/Mood:
Cravings/Appetite:	Health:

Date:	Energy/Mood:
Cravings/Appetite:	Health:

Date:	Energy/Mood:
Cravings/Appetite:	Health:

Notes:

Your baby's head may drop down into your pelvis now, in preparation for birth, but there's still plenty of time.

week 38

Hopefully you will start finding it easier to breathe now if your baby has dropped lower into your pelvis. But the need to urinate frequently may be back with a vengeance!

How am I feeling this week?

Date:	Energy:
Mood:	Appetite:
Cravings:	Health:

Date:	Energy:
Mood:	Appetite:
Cravings:	Health:

Date:	Energy:
Mood:	Appetite:
Cravings:	Health:

Date:	Energy:
Mood:	Appetite:
Cravings:	Health:

week 38

Date:	Energy:
Mood:	Appetite:
Cravings:	Health:

Date:	Energy:
Mood:	Appetite:
Cravings:	Health:

Date:	Energy:
Mood:	Appetite:
Cravings:	Health:

Notes:

Your baby is now a good size and weight. She is ready to be born.

week 39

At this time of your pregnancy, you may notice a sudden urge to clean and tidy your home. This is your nesting instinct coming into play to make sure everything is ready for the baby's arrival. Don't overdo it and accept all offers of help!

THINGS to do
• If you are using a TENS machine for pain relief, have a few more practice runs with it first.

How am I feeling this week?

Date:	Energy:
Mood:	Appetite:
Cravings:	Health:
Date:	Energy:
Mood:	Appetite:
Cravings:	Health:
Date:	Energy:
Mood:	Appetite:
Cravings:	Health:

week 39

Date:	Energy/Mood:
Cravings/Appetite:	Health:

Date:	Energy/Mood:
Cravings/Appetite:	Health:

Date:	Energy/Mood:
Cravings/Appetite:	Health:

Date:	Energy/Mood:
Cravings/Appetite:	Health:

Notes:

The bones in your baby's skull are able to slide over each other and overlap so his head can pass through the birth canal without being damaged.

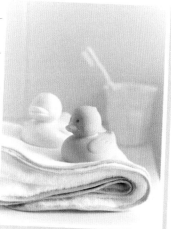

week 40

After a nine-month wait, your due week has finally arrived! However, as only 5 per cent of babies are actually born on their due date, don't be surprised if yours doesn't stick to the schedule!

How am I feeling this week?

Date:	Energy:
Mood:	Appetite:
Cravings:	Health:

Date:	Energy:
Mood:	Appetite:
Cravings:	Health:

Date:	Energy:
Mood:	Appetite:
Cravings:	Health:

Date:	Energy:
Mood:	Appetite:
Cravings:	Health:

week 40

Date: Energy/Mood:

Cravings/Appetite: Health:

Date: Energy/Mood:

Cravings/Appetite: Health:

Date: Energy/Mood:

Cravings/Appetite: Health:

Notes:

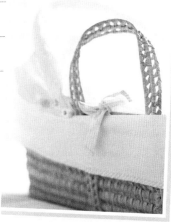

A baby has no functioning tear ducts for the first couple of weeks — during this time her first cries will be tearless.

153

week 41

You're now overdue but try not to be too fed up – this is quite common, especially for a first-time mother. Use the extra time to relax, watch television, read a book, see friends and generally look after yourself.

COPING with the situation

• If your telephone constantly rings with people eager to find out if you've given birth yet, it might be a good idea to record an answering machine message to explain what stage you're at. This will prevent you from getting too frustrated with having to keep answering the phone and saying the same thing. Alternatively, you could send a group text message or email.

How do I feel now I'm overdue?

How am I feeling this week?

Date:	Energy:
Mood:	Appetite:
Cravings:	Health:

Date:	Energy:
Mood:	Appetite:
Cravings:	Health:

week 41

Date:	Energy:
Mood:	Appetite:
Cravings:	Health:
Date:	Energy:
Mood:	Appetite:
Cravings:	Health:
Date:	Energy:
Mood:	Appetite:
Cravings:	Health:
Date:	Energy:
Mood:	Appetite:
Cravings:	Health:
Date:	Energy/Mood:
Cravings/Appetite:	Health:

week 42

The end is in sight – your baby is likely to be born this week. Read up about being induced so you are prepared for this should your baby still not want to come out of his own accord.

How do I feel now I am still overdue?

_____

_____

_____

How am I feeling this week?

Date:	Energy:
Mood:	Appetite:
Cravings:	Health:

Date:	Energy:
Mood:	Appetite:
Cravings:	Health:

Date:	Energy:
Mood:	Appetite:
Cravings:	Health:

week 42

Date:	Energy/Mood:
Cravings/Appetite:	Health:

Date:	Energy/Mood:
Cravings/Appetite:	Health:

Date:	Energy/Mood:
Cravings/Appetite:	Health:

Date:	Energy/Mood:
Cravings/Appetite:	Health:

Notes:

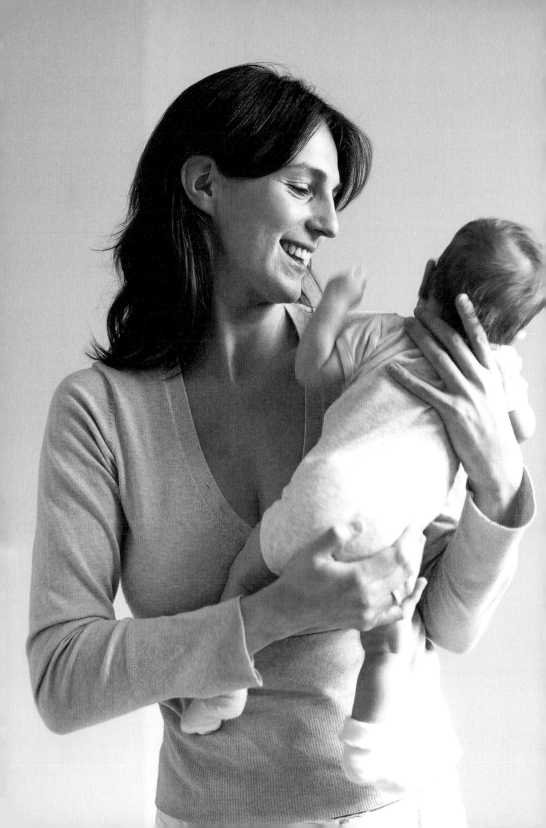

labour & birth

You're almost there – very soon you'll be holding your precious
newborn in your arms. In the final weeks of pregnancy, planning
for labour and birth – from writing a birth plan to packing your
hospital bag – will help you to stay calm and in control.

countdown to D-Day

As your due date approaches you are bound to be anxious and think that you are running out of time. Write down your feelings and your to-do list here and try to stay calm!

Feelings:

countdown to D-Day

To-do list:

birth plan

Writing a birth plan is a useful way to think about the type of birth you would like and make some sensible decisions before those labour pains begin. Below are some things to consider.

Who is your ideal birth partner?

Who is your back-up birth partner?

Do you want to be induced?

Would you be against a Caesarean delivery?

birth plan

What is your preferred method of pain relief, if any?

Do you want a water birth?

Do you have a preferred birthing position?

Would you prefer an episiotomy or natural tear?

birth plan

Do you want your partner to cut the umbilical cord?

_____

_____

_____

Would you like to breastfeed straight away?

_____

_____

_____

Do you want to deliver the placenta naturally?

_____

_____

_____

Do you have any special requests?

_____

_____

_____

_____

birth plan

Notes:
_____

_____

_____

_____

_____

_____

_____

_____

_____

_____

_____

_____

_____

_____

_____

_____

_____

_____

_____

packing your hospital bag

You'll probably feel calmer once your hospital bag is packed and positioned at the front door for a quick exit! Below are some useful items to include.

My hospital bag checklist

For me

☐ Birth plan

☐ Old T-shirt/nightdress for birth

☐ Socks

☐ Slippers

☐ Water spray (to cool me down)

☐ Mirror (if I want to see the baby being born)

☐ Flannels and towels

☐ Camera/video

☐ Toiletries

☐ Tissues

☐ Hot water bottle

☐ Front-opening nightdress

☐ Dressing gown

☐ 2-3 maternity/nursing bras

☐ Snacks for me/my partner

☐ Music/magazines/playing cards

☐ Coins for pay phone

☐ Disposable knickers

☐ Maternity sanitary towels

☐ Breast pads

☐ Coming home clothes

Extra items

☐

☐

Notes:

packing your hospital bag

For baby	Additional items for a home birth
☐ 2–3 sleepsuits	☐ Pillows or large cushions
☐ 2–3 vests	☐ Lamp or bright torch
☐ Scratch mittens	☐ Clean sheets
☐ Shawl/blanket	☐ Plastic sheeting
☐ Hat	☐ Hot water and soap
☐ Nappies/diapers	☐ Rubbish/trash bags
☐ Cotton wool	Extra items
☐ Cream - zinc & castor oil/Vaseline	☐
☐ Car seat	☐
Extra items	☐
☐	
☐	
☐	

Notes:

announcing the birth

There are now so many different ways of contacting people that it can help to think about how you'll inform people about the birth.

	Name	Contact number
Phone immediately:		

	Name	Contact number
Phone later:		

announcing the birth

	Name	Contact number
Send text message:		

	Name	Email address
Send email:		

record of your labour

When the dust has settled, you might want to take some time to think about your labour and birth experience and make some notes.

My labour started at: on:

I went into hospital at: on:

I went to hospital by:

When I arrived at the hospital:

How I felt at this stage:

My baby was delivered at: on:

I was in labour for: hours: minutes:

record of your labour

What pain relief did I use?

Who was present at the birth?

Who cut the baby's umbilical cord?

Did the baby cry straight away?

Was childbirth how I imagined it to be?

Notes:

record of your labour

In what ways was it different?

_____

_____

_____

If I did it all over again would I change anything?

_____

_____

_____

How do I feel now our baby is born?

_____

_____

_____

How does my partner feel now our baby is born?

_____

_____

_____

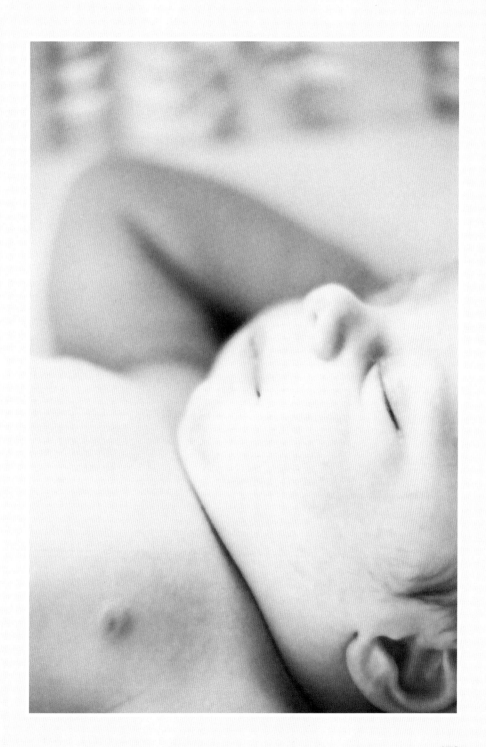

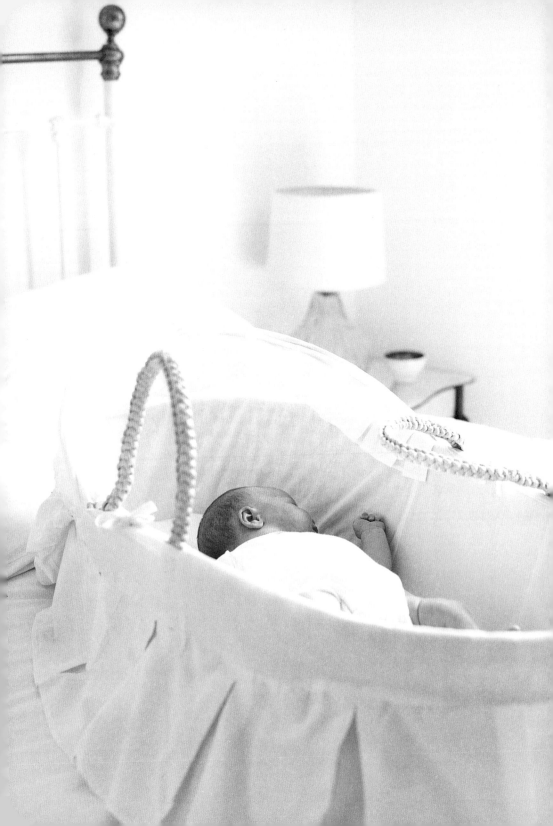

the early weeks

Elated but exhausted, you may barely remember anything
of the first few weeks. Use these pages to write down those
all-important details about your newborn and stay organized
with gift lists and feeding logs.

about my baby

Record the important details of your baby's birth and note down how you felt on that very special day.

Name:

Date of birth: | Time of birth:

Weight: | Length:

Hair colour: | Eye colour:

Hospital:

Name of midwife:

Notes:

First 24 hours:

about my baby

Stick your first photos here of your new baby

gifts received

While it's lovely to receive gifts for your newborn, it can be overwhelming in those whirlwind first weeks. Keep a note of who has sent what as you receive each gift.

Gift:	Gift:
From:	From:
Thank you card sent?	Thank you card sent?
Gift:	Gift:
From:	From:
Thank you card sent?	Thank you card sent?
Gift:	Gift:
From:	From:
Thank you card sent?	Thank you card sent?
Gift:	Gift:
From:	From:
Thank you card sent?	Thank you card sent?

gifts received

Gift:

From:

Thank you card sent?

Gift:

From:

Thank you card sent?

Gift:

From:

Thank you card sent?

Gift:

From:

Thank you card sent?

Gift:

From:

Thank you card sent?

Gift:

From:

Thank you card sent?

Notes:

feeding log

Whether you're breast- or bottle-feeding your baby, it's useful to keep a record of milk intake in those all-important first few weeks of life and to gradually establish a feeding routine.

Breastfeeding

Date	Time	Length of feed (right)	Length of feed (left)

feeding log

Breastfeeding

Date	Time	Length of feed (right)	Length of feed (left)

feeding log

Combination feeding

Date	Time	Length of breastfeed	Amount of bottle-feed (ml/fl oz.)

feeding log

Bottle-feeding

Date	Time	Amount of bottle-feed(ml/fl oz.)

postnatal appointments

Use this space to jot down the details of any medical appointments you might attend after the birth of your baby along with any useful advice you were given.

Date: Time:

Advice:

Date: Time:

Advice:

Date: Time:

Advice:

Date: Time:

Advice:

postnatal appointments

Date: Time:

Advice:

Date: Time:

Advice:

Date: Time:

Advice:

Date: Time:

Advice:

Date: Time:

Advice:

to-do list

to-do list

additional notes

additional notes

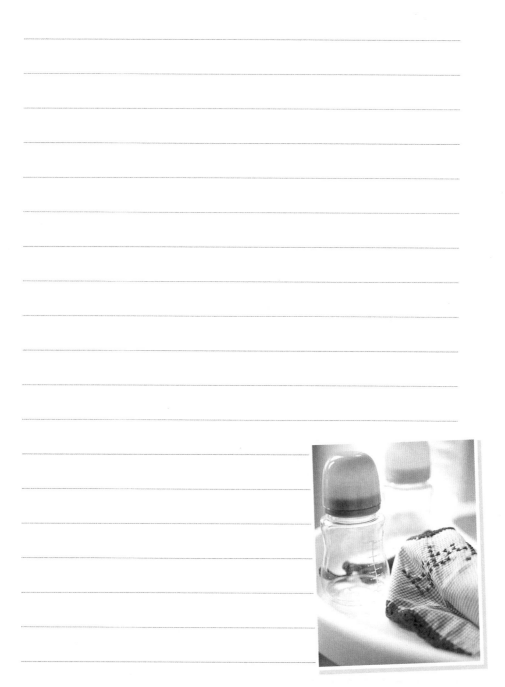

useful organizations

There is a wealth of information online to guide you through your pregnancy and the first few months of parenthood. Here are a few suggested websites but also keep a note of any others you find useful.

Action on Pre-Eclampsia (APEC): www.apec.org.uk

Username: Password:

Active Birth Centre: www.activebirthcentre.com

Username: Password:

Association for Improvement in Maternity Services (AIMS):
www.aims.org.uk

Username: Password:

BabyCentre: www.babycentre.com

Username: Password:

The Breastfeeding Network: www.breastfeedingnetwork.org.uk

Username: Password:

useful organizations

the Bump: www.thebump.com

Username: Password:

La Leche League: www.laleche.org.uk

Username: Password:

NCT (National Childbirth Trust): www.nct.org.uk

Username: Password:

Net Mums: www.netmums.com

Username   Password

Others:

acknowledgements/credits

Thanks to the team at RPS, especially Julia Charles for the opportunity to write this journal and Nathan Joyce for editing it. Thanks to my good friend Debs, who cleverly got pregnant at the same time as me. You helped me to stay calm and organized throughout my pregnancy and have been helpful and inspirational ever since.

Photography credits

Peter Cassidy
Page 147

Carolyn Barber
Pages 41, 51

Dan Duchars
Pages 91, 125, 127, 158, 171

Chris Everard
Pages 17, 81
Winfried Heinze
Pages 10, 14, 62, 65, 88, 121, 122, 157

Debi Treloar
Pages 3, 4, 23, 27, 37, 61, 87, 97, 98, 138, 153, 167, 173, 189

Kate Whitaker
Page 75

Penny Wincer
Page 35

Polly Wreford
Pages 2, 30, 33, 45, 46, 49, 54, 111, 151, 174, 179